This Food and Exercise Journal Belongs to

_____

"The difference between your body this week and next week is what you do for the next seven days to achieve your goals."

Exercise Journal For My Week

Date	Exercise	Reps	Sets

Food and Exercise Journal Notes for week:

Food Journal For My Week

Date	Breakfast	Lunch	Dinner	Snacks	Total
Mon					
Calories					
Tues					
Calories					
Wed					
Calories					
Thurs					
Calories					
Fri					
Calories					
Sat					
Calories					
Sun					
Calories					

Food and Exercise Journal Notes for week:

Workout Journal For My Week

Date	Exercise	Reps	Sets

Food and Exercise Journal Notes for week:

Food Journal For My Week

Date	Breakfast	Lunch	Dinner	Snacks	Total
Mon					
Calories					
Tues					
Calories					
Wed					
Calories					
Thurs					
Calories					
Fri					
Calories					
Sat					
Calories					
Sun					
Calories					

Food and Exercise Journal Notes for week:

Workout Journal For My Week

Date	Exercise	Reps	Sets

Food and Exercise Journal Notes for week:

Food Journal For My Week

Date	Breakfast	Lunch	Dinner	Snacks	Total
Mon					
Calories					
Tues					
Calories					
Wed					
Calories					
Thurs					
Calories					
Fri					
Calories					
Sat					
Calories					
Sun					
Calories					

Food and Exercise Journal Notes for week:

Workout Journal For My Week

Date	Exercise	Reps	Sets

Food and Exercise Journal Notes for week:

Food Journal For My Week

Date	Breakfast	Lunch	Dinner	Snacks	Total
Mon					
Calories					
Tues					
Calories					
Wed					
Calories					
Thurs					
Calories					
Fri					
Calories					
Sat					
Calories					
Sun					
Calories					

Food and Exercise Journal Notes for week:

Workout Journal For My Week

Date	Exercise	Reps	Sets

Food and Exercise Journal Notes for week:

Food Journal For My Week

Date	Breakfast	Lunch	Dinner	Snacks	Total
Mon					
Calories					
Tues					
Calories					
Wed					
Calories					
Thurs					
Calories					
Fri					
Calories					
Sat					
Calories					
Sun					
Calories					

Food and Exercise Journal Notes for week:

Workout Journal For My Week

Date	Exercise	Reps	Sets

Food and Exercise Journal Notes for week:

Food Journal For My Week

Date	Breakfast	Lunch	Dinner	Snacks	Total
Mon					
Calories					
Tues					
Calories					
Wed					
Calories					
Thurs					
Calories					
Fri					
Calories					
Sat					
Calories					
Sun					
Calories					

Food and Exercise Journal Notes for week:

Workout Journal For My Week

Date	Exercise	Reps	Sets

Food and Exercise Journal Notes for week:

Food Journal For My Week

Date	Breakfast	Lunch	Dinner	Snacks	Total
Mon					
Calories					
Tues					
Calories					
Wed					
Calories					
Thurs					
Calories					
Fri					
Calories					
Sat					
Calories					
Sun					
Calories					

Food and Exercise Journal Notes for week:

Workout Journal For My Week

Date	Exercise	Reps	Sets

Food and Exercise Journal Notes for week:

Food Journal For My Week

Date	Breakfast	Lunch	Dinner	Snacks	Total
Mon					
Calories					
Tues					
Calories					
Wed					
Calories					
Thurs					
Calories					
Fri					
Calories					
Sat					
Calories					
Sun					
Calories					

Food and Exercise Journal Notes for week:

Workout Journal For My Week

Date	Exercise	Reps	Sets

Food and Exercise Journal Notes for week:

Food Journal For My Week

Date	Breakfast	Lunch	Dinner	Snacks	Total
Mon					
Calories					
Tues					
Calories					
Wed					
Calories					
Thurs					
Calories					
Fri					
Calories					
Sat					
Calories					
Sun					
Calories					

Food and Exercise Journal Notes for week:

Workout Journal For My Week

Date	Exercise	Reps	Sets

Notes for week:

Food Journal For My Week

Date	Breakfast	Lunch	Dinner	Snacks	Total
Mon					
Calories					
Tues					
Calories					
Wed					
Calories					
Thurs					
Calories					
Fri					
Calories					
Sat					
Calories					
Sun					
Calories					

Notes for week:

Workout Journal For My Week

Date	Exercise	Reps	Sets

Notes for week:

Food Journal For My Week

Date	Breakfast	Lunch	Dinner	Snacks	Total
Mon					
Calories					
Tues					
Calories					
Wed					
Calories					
Thurs					
Calories					
Fri					
Calories					
Sat					
Calories					
Sun					
Calories					

Notes for week:

Workout Journal For My Week

Date	Exercise	Reps	Sets

Notes for week:

Food Journal For My Week

Date	Breakfast	Lunch	Dinner	Snacks	Total
Mon					
Calories					
Tues					
Calories					
Wed					
Calories					
Thurs					
Calories					
Fri					
Calories					
Sat					
Calories					
Sun					
Calories					

Notes for week:

Workout Journal For My Week

Date	Exercise	Reps	Sets

Notes for week:

Food Journal For My Week

Date	Breakfast	Lunch	Dinner	Snacks	Total
Mon					
Calories					
Tues					
Calories					
Wed					
Calories					
Thurs					
Calories					
Fri					
Calories					
Sat					
Calories					
Sun					
Calories					

Notes for week:

Workout Journal For My Week

Date	Exercise	Reps	Sets

Notes for week:

Food Journal For My Week

Date	Breakfast	Lunch	Dinner	Snacks	Total
Mon					
Calories					
Tues					
Calories					
Wed					
Calories					
Thurs					
Calories					
Fri					
Calories					
Sat					
Calories					
Sun					
Calories					

Notes for week:

Workout Journal For My Week

Date	Exercise	Reps	Sets

Notes for week:

Food Journal For My Week

Date	Breakfast	Lunch	Dinner	Snacks	Total
Mon					
Calories					
Tues					
Calories					
Wed					
Calories					
Thurs					
Calories					
Fri					
Calories					
Sat					
Calories					
Sun					
Calories					

Notes for week:

Workout Journal For My Week

Date	Exercise	Reps	Sets

Notes for week:

Food Journal For My Week

Date	Breakfast	Lunch	Dinner	Snacks	Total
Mon					
Calories					
Tues					
Calories					
Wed					
Calories					
Thurs					
Calories					
Fri					
Calories					
Sat					
Calories					
Sun					
Calories					

Notes for week:

Workout Journal For My Week

Date	Exercise	Reps	Sets

Notes for week:

Food Journal For My Week

Date	Breakfast	Lunch	Dinner	Snacks	Total
Mon					
Calories					
Tues					
Calories					
Wed					
Calories					
Thurs					
Calories					
Fri					
Calories					
Sat					
Calories					
Sun					
Calories					

Notes for week:

Workout Journal For My Week

Date	Exercise	Reps	Sets

Notes for week:

Food Journal For My Week

Date	Breakfast	Lunch	Dinner	Snacks	Total
Mon					
Calories					
Tues					
Calories					
Wed					
Calories					
Thurs					
Calories					
Fri					
Calories					
Sat					
Calories					
Sun					
Calories					

Notes for week:

Workout Journal For My Week

Date	Exercise	Reps	Sets

Notes for week:

Food Journal For My Week

Date	Breakfast	Lunch	Dinner	Snacks	Total
Mon					
Calories					
Tues					
Calories					
Wed					
Calories					
Thurs					
Calories					
Fri					
Calories					
Sat					
Calories					
Sun					
Calories					

Notes for week:

Workout Journal For My Week

Date	Exercise	Reps	Sets

Notes for week:

Food Journal For My Week

Date	Breakfast	Lunch	Dinner	Snacks	Total
Mon					
Calories					
Tues					
Calories					
Wed					
Calories					
Thurs					
Calories					
Fri					
Calories					
Sat					
Calories					
Sun					
Calories					

Notes for week:

Workout Journal For My Week

Date	Exercise	Reps	Sets

Notes for week:

Food Journal For My Week

Date	Breakfast	Lunch	Dinner	Snacks	Total
Mon					
Calories					
Tues					
Calories					
Wed					
Calories					
Thurs					
Calories					
Fri					
Calories					
Sat					
Calories					
Sun					
Calories					

Notes for week:

Workout Journal For My Week

Date	Exercise	Reps	Sets

Notes for week:

Food Journal For My Week

Date	Breakfast	Lunch	Dinner	Snacks	Total
Mon					
Calories					
Tues					
Calories					
Wed					
Calories					
Thurs					
Calories					
Fri					
Calories					
Sat					
Calories					
Sun					
Calories					

Notes for week:

Workout Journal For My Week

Date	Exercise	Reps	Sets

Notes for week:

Food Journal For My Week

Date	Breakfast	Lunch	Dinner	Snacks	Total
Mon					
Calories					
Tues					
Calories					
Wed					
Calories					
Thurs					
Calories					
Fri					
Calories					
Sat					
Calories					
Sun					
Calories					

Notes for week:

Workout Journal For My Week

Date	Exercise	Reps	Sets

Notes for week:

Food Journal For My Week

Date	Breakfast	Lunch	Dinner	Snacks	Total
Mon					
Calories					
Tues					
Calories					
Wed					
Calories					
Thurs					
Calories					
Fri					
Calories					
Sat					
Calories					
Sun					
Calories					

Notes for week:

Workout Journal For My Week

Date	Exercise	Reps	Sets

Notes for week:

Food Journal For My Week

Date	Breakfast	Lunch	Dinner	Snacks	Total
Mon					
Calories					
Tues					
Calories					
Wed					
Calories					
Thurs					
Calories					
Fri					
Calories					
Sat					
Calories					
Sun					
Calories					

Notes for week:

Workout Journal For My Week

Date	Exercise	Reps	Sets

Notes for week:

Food Journal For My Week

Date	Breakfast	Lunch	Dinner	Snacks	Total
Mon					
Calories					
Tues					
Calories					
Wed					
Calories					
Thurs					
Calories					
Fri					
Calories					
Sat					
Calories					
Sun					
Calories					

Notes for week:

Workout Journal For My Week

Date	Exercise	Reps	Sets

Notes for week:

Food Journal For My Week

Date	Breakfast	Lunch	Dinner	Snacks	Total
Mon					
Calories					
Tues					
Calories					
Wed					
Calories					
Thurs					
Calories					
Fri					
Calories					
Sat					
Calories					
Sun					
Calories					

Notes for week:

Workout Journal For My Week

Date	Exercise	Reps	Sets

Notes for week:

Food Journal For My Week

Date	Breakfast	Lunch	Dinner	Snacks	Total
Mon					
Calories					
Tues					
Calories					
Wed					
Calories					
Thurs					
Calories					
Fri					
Calories					
Sat					
Calories					
Sun					
Calories					

Notes for week:

Workout Journal For My Week

Date	Exercise	Reps	Sets

Notes for week:

Food Journal For My Week

Date	Breakfast	Lunch	Dinner	Snacks	Total
Mon					
Calories					
Tues					
Calories					
Wed					
Calories					
Thurs					
Calories					
Fri					
Calories					
Sat					
Calories					
Sun					
Calories					

Notes for week:

Workout Journal For My Week

Date	Exercise	Reps	Sets

Notes for week:

Food Journal For My Week

Date	Breakfast	Lunch	Dinner	Snacks	Total
Mon					
Calories					
Tues					
Calories					
Wed					
Calories					
Thurs					
Calories					
Fri					
Calories					
Sat					
Calories					
Sun					
Calories					

Notes for week:

Workout Journal For My Week

Date	Exercise	Reps	Sets

Notes for week:

Food Journal For My Week

Date	Breakfast	Lunch	Dinner	Snacks	Total
Mon					
Calories					
Tues					
Calories					
Wed					
Calories					
Thurs					
Calories					
Fri					
Calories					
Sat					
Calories					
Sun					
Calories					

Notes for week:

Workout Journal For My Week

Date	Exercise	Reps	Sets

Notes for week:

Food Journal For My Week

Date	Breakfast	Lunch	Dinner	Snacks	Total
Mon					
Calories					
Tues					
Calories					
Wed					
Calories					
Thurs					
Calories					
Fri					
Calories					
Sat					
Calories					
Sun					
Calories					

Notes for week:

Workout Journal For My Week

Date	Exercise	Reps	Sets

Notes for week:

Food Journal For My Week

Date	Breakfast	Lunch	Dinner	Snacks	Total
Mon					
Calories					
Tues					
Calories					
Wed					
Calories					
Thurs					
Calories					
Fri					
Calories					
Sat					
Calories					
Sun					
Calories					

Notes for week:

Workout Journal For My Week

Date	Exercise	Reps	Sets

Notes for week:

Food Journal For My Week

Date	Breakfast	Lunch	Dinner	Snacks	Total
Mon					
Calories					
Tues					
Calories					
Wed					
Calories					
Thurs					
Calories					
Fri					
Calories					
Sat					
Calories					
Sun					
Calories					

Notes for week:

Workout Journal For My Week

Date	Exercise	Reps	Sets

Notes for week:

Food Journal For My Week

Date	Breakfast	Lunch	Dinner	Snacks	Total
Mon					
Calories					
Tues					
Calories					
Wed					
Calories					
Thurs					
Calories					
Fri					
Calories					
Sat					
Calories					
Sun					
Calories					

Notes for week:

Workout Journal For My Week

Date	Exercise	Reps	Sets

Notes for week:

Food Journal For My Week

Date	Breakfast	Lunch	Dinner	Snacks	Total
Mon					
Calories					
Tues					
Calories					
Wed					
Calories					
Thurs					
Calories					
Fri					
Calories					
Sat					
Calories					
Sun					
Calories					

Notes for week:

Workout Journal For My Week

Date	Exercise	Reps	Sets

Notes for week:

Food Journal For My Week

Date	Breakfast	Lunch	Dinner	Snacks	Total
Mon					
Calories					
Tues					
Calories					
Wed					
Calories					
Thurs					
Calories					
Fri					
Calories					
Sat					
Calories					
Sun					
Calories					

Notes for week:

Workout Journal For My Week

Date	Exercise	Reps	Sets

Notes for week:

Food Journal For My Week

Date	Breakfast	Lunch	Dinner	Snacks	Total
Mon					
Calories					
Tues					
Calories					
Wed					
Calories					
Thurs					
Calories					
Fri					
Calories					
Sat					
Calories					
Sun					
Calories					

Notes for week:

Workout Journal For My Week

Date	Exercise	Reps	Sets

Notes for week:

Food Journal For My Week

Date	Breakfast	Lunch	Dinner	Snacks	Total
Mon					
Calories					
Tues					
Calories					
Wed					
Calories					
Thurs					
Calories					
Fri					
Calories					
Sat					
Calories					
Sun					
Calories					

Notes for week:

Workout Journal For My Week

Date	Exercise	Reps	Sets

Notes for week:

Food Journal For My Week

Date	Breakfast	Lunch	Dinner	Snacks	Total
Mon					
Calories					
Tues					
Calories					
Wed					
Calories					
Thurs					
Calories					
Fri					
Calories					
Sat					
Calories					
Sun					
Calories					

Notes for week:

Workout Journal For My Week

Date	Exercise	Reps	Sets

Notes for week:

Food Journal For My Week

Date	Breakfast	Lunch	Dinner	Snacks	Total
Mon					
Calories					
Tues					
Calories					
Wed					
Calories					
Thurs					
Calories					
Fri					
Calories					
Sat					
Calories					
Sun					
Calories					

Notes for week:

Workout Journal For My Week

Date	Exercise	Reps	Sets

Notes for week:

Food Journal For My Week

Date	Breakfast	Lunch	Dinner	Snacks	Total
Mon					
Calories					
Tues					
Calories					
Wed					
Calories					
Thurs					
Calories					
Fri					
Calories					
Sat					
Calories					
Sun					
Calories					

Notes for week:

Workout Journal For My Week

Date	Exercise	Reps	Sets

Notes for week:

Food Journal For My Week

Date	Breakfast	Lunch	Dinner	Snacks	Total
Mon					
Calories					
Tues					
Calories					
Wed					
Calories					
Thurs					
Calories					
Fri					
Calories					
Sat					
Calories					
Sun					
Calories					

Notes for week:

Workout Journal For My Week

Date	Exercise	Reps	Sets

Notes for week:

Food Journal For My Week

Date	Breakfast	Lunch	Dinner	Snacks	Total
Mon					
Calories					
Tues					
Calories					
Wed					
Calories					
Thurs					
Calories					
Fri					
Calories					
Sat					
Calories					
Sun					
Calories					

Notes for week:

Workout Journal For My Week

Date	Exercise	Reps	Sets

Notes for week:

Food Journal For My Week

Date	Breakfast	Lunch	Dinner	Snacks	Total
Mon					
Calories					
Tues					
Calories					
Wed					
Calories					
Thurs					
Calories					
Fri					
Calories					
Sat					
Calories					
Sun					
Calories					

Notes for week:

Workout Journal For My Week

Date	Exercise	Reps	Sets

Notes for week:

Food Journal For My Week

Date	Breakfast	Lunch	Dinner	Snacks	Total
Mon					
Calories					
Tues					
Calories					
Wed					
Calories					
Thurs					
Calories					
Fri					
Calories					
Sat					
Calories					
Sun					
Calories					

Notes for week:

Workout Journal For My Week

Date	Exercise	Reps	Sets

Notes for week:

Food Journal For My Week

Date	Breakfast	Lunch	Dinner	Snacks	Total
Mon					
Calories					
Tues					
Calories					
Wed					
Calories					
Thurs					
Calories					
Fri					
Calories					
Sat					
Calories					
Sun					
Calories					

Notes for week:

Workout Journal For My Week

Date	Exercise	Reps	Sets

Notes for week:

Food Journal For My Week

Date	Breakfast	Lunch	Dinner	Snacks	Total
Mon					
Calories					
Tues					
Calories					
Wed					
Calories					
Thurs					
Calories					
Fri					
Calories					
Sat					
Calories					
Sun					
Calories					

Notes for week:

Workout Journal For My Week

Date	Exercise	Reps	Sets

Notes for week:

Food Journal For My Week

Date	Breakfast	Lunch	Dinner	Snacks	Total
Mon					
Calories					
Tues					
Calories					
Wed					
Calories					
Thurs					
Calories					
Fri					
Calories					
Sat					
Calories					
Sun					
Calories					

Notes for week:

Workout Journal For My Week

Date	Exercise	Reps	Sets

Notes for week:

Food Journal For My Week

Date	Breakfast	Lunch	Dinner	Snacks	Total
Mon					
Calories					
Tues					
Calories					
Wed					
Calories					
Thurs					
Calories					
Fri					
Calories					
Sat					
Calories					
Sun					
Calories					

Notes for week:

Workout Journal For My Week

Date	Exercise	Reps	Sets

Notes for week:

Food Journal For My Week

Date	Breakfast	Lunch	Dinner	Snacks	Total
Mon					
Calories					
Tues					
Calories					
Wed					
Calories					
Thurs					
Calories					
Fri					
Calories					
Sat					
Calories					
Sun					
Calories					

Notes for week:

Workout Journal For My Week

Date	Exercise	Reps	Sets

Notes for week:

Food Journal For My Week

Date	Breakfast	Lunch	Dinner	Snacks	Total
Mon					
Calories					
Tues					
Calories					
Wed					
Calories					
Thurs					
Calories					
Fri					
Calories					
Sat					
Calories					
Sun					
Calories					

Notes for week:

Workout Journal For My Week

Date	Exercise	Reps	Sets

Notes for week:

Food Journal For My Week

Date	Breakfast	Lunch	Dinner	Snacks	Total
Mon					
Calories					
Tues					
Calories					
Wed					
Calories					
Thurs					
Calories					
Fri					
Calories					
Sat					
Calories					
Sun					
Calories					

Notes for week:

Workout Journal For My Week

Date	Exercise	Reps	Sets

Notes for week:

Food Journal For My Week

Date	Breakfast	Lunch	Dinner	Snacks	Total
Mon					
Calories					
Tues					
Calories					
Wed					
Calories					
Thurs					
Calories					
Fri					
Calories					
Sat					
Calories					
Sun					
Calories					

Notes for week:

Workout Journal For My Week

Date	Exercise	Reps	Sets

Notes for week:

Food Journal For My Week

Date	Breakfast	Lunch	Dinner	Snacks	Total
Mon					
Calories					
Tues					
Calories					
Wed					
Calories					
Thurs					
Calories					
Fri					
Calories					
Sat					
Calories					
Sun					
Calories					

Notes for week:

Workout Journal For My Week

Date	Exercise	Reps	Sets

Notes for week:

Food Journal For My Week

Date	Breakfast	Lunch	Dinner	Snacks	Total
Mon					
Calories					
Tues					
Calories					
Wed					
Calories					
Thurs					
Calories					
Fri					
Calories					
Sat					
Calories					
Sun					
Calories					

Notes for week:

www.ingramcontent.com/pod-product-compliance
Lightning Source LLC
Chambersburg PA
CBHW070118290526
45789CB00005B/2059